BEATING A-FIB

A Natural Approach to Atrial Fibrillation

By

Lisa M White

Introduction

What is Atrial Fibrillation?

Clotting and Stroke Risk.

Conventional Treatments for Afib

Recognised Causes of A-fib

Inflammation and A-fib

Treating A-fib By Reducing Inflammation.

   Tackle Food Intolerances And Trigger Foods

   Trigger Foods

   Aspartame

   Salt

   Dairy Products

   Sugar

Resolve Magnesium Deficiency

   Symptoms of a Magnesium Deficiency

   Resolving Magnesium Deficiency.

   Magnesium Rich Foods

   Transdermal Magnesium

   Magnesium Overdose

Treat low level infection.

   H-Pylori

   Eradicating H-Pylori

The effect of mastic gum on Helicobacter pylori: a randomized pilot study.

Don't Be Sedentary

Treat Sleep Apnea

Weight Loss and Afib

An Ideal Diet for A-Fib?

Reduce stress

Acupuncture/Acupressure

Yoga

   Energy Breath (Bellows Breath/Stimulating Breath)

   Relaxing Breath

Chiropractic Adjustment

EFT Emotional Freedom Technique

   Basic EFT technique.

Toward A More Positive Future

My A-Fib Story and How I Cured Myself

Introduction

If you have a-fib you are not alone. One in ten people will suffer at least one atrial fibrillation attack in their lifetime. Whilst an a-fib attack can be extremely frightening, it is not generally regarded as life threatening.

For some people, the cause of their a-fib is apparent. A-fib commonly accompanies heart disease, thyroid problems and high blood pressure. It can occur sporadically after over indulgence in alcohol – the "holiday heart" syndrome or at times of stress. Several studies have now proved the link between obesity and atrial fibrillation.

For other people, the cause of their atrial fibrillation is a mystery. Around 10-15% of cases of atrial fibrillation occur when there is no apparent heart disease or any other obvious risk factor. This is known as "lone atrial fibrillation".

Whatever the underlying cause of your atrial fibrillation, it is important to work with your doctor to formulate a treatment strategy to suit your individual circumstances and triggers. This book is not a substitute for qualified medical advice, so please consult with your doctor prior to trying anything new. This is particularly important if you have heart disease or if you are taking blood thinners.

I personally cured my own lone a-fib with no surgery and no drugs and have now been free of attacks for several years. After a great deal of research and detective work I found that the underlying cause in my case was a chronic mineral deficiency. Other patients I have met have greatly improved their condition by avoiding certain foods or losing weight. With a-fib there is no cure-all or plan to suit everybody, it is a case of working with your doctors and listening to your body to find out what works for you.

Try to find the ideal balance between medical management and self-help. Learning as much as you can about the condition will not only help to offset your fear, it will also empower you. A-fib can be a scary condition, particularly during an acute attack but if you understand what is happening, the fear will subside. Educating yourself will also allow you to communicate more effectively with your doctors and be more pro-active in your own care.

Firstly, let's look at what a-fib is and how it occurs.

What is Atrial Fibrillation?

Atrial fibrillation is a very common arrhythmia, the medical term used for a heart which is beating irregularly or out of rhythm. The human heart normally beats in a smooth organised way at a rate of between 60-100 beats per minute. When atrial fibrillation or a-fib for short occurs, the electrical signals which usually provide a regular heartbeat get disrupted. This means that the heart starts to beat out of rhythm and faster, sometimes up to 180 beats per minute or more.

Doctors sometimes refer to the heart rhythm during an a-fib attack as "irregularly irregular". If you feel your pulse during an episode you will find there is no regular pattern to it – there may be missed beats, rapid beats, runs and pauses. It is like a marching band totally out of sync.

Whilst this may seem like a medical emergency, in most cases it is not. In fact, the disordered signals occur in the top part of the heart – the atria, only account for about 25% of the heart's pumping capacity.

Some people have no symptoms at all during an a-fib attack, it is sometimes only discovered on a routine check-up. Other people may have violent palpitations, fatigue, shortness of breath, dizziness, chest pain or reduced exercise tolerance.

How Your Heart Beats.

The heart consists of four chambers. The top part of the heart is called the atria and the bottom part of the heart is the ventricles. Normally, when the heart beats, an electrical signal travels in an ordered fashion from the top to the bottom of the heart. This makes the heart contract and blood is pumped around the body.

In the right atrium at the top of the heart, there is a node called the sinoatrial (SA) node. This is responsible for initiating a heartbeat. Each heartbeat starts in the SA node and then travels to another node – the AV node which is in the middle of the heart. This node slows and regulates the heart beat impulse before it passes down to the ventricles. During the slowing phase, the ventricles fill with blood. Once the signal moves downwards it forces the ventricles to contract, pumping out blood. Once the ventricles are empty, the sequence begins again.

What Happens During A-fib?

A-fib occurs when the heart beat starts in a different part of the heart, usually around the pulmonary veins. When this happens, instead of a nice regular heartbeat, the electrical system misfires and floods the atria with impulses. It is a bit like a dam breaking, instead of everything flowing in an orderly manner, impulses rush everywhere causing the atria to rapidly twitch or fibrillate up to 600 times a minute.

Luckily, not all these signals are passed down to the ventricles as the AV node cannot keep pace. If it could, the heart would try to beat between 300 and 600 times per minute. Instead, the AV node passes only some of the signals down to the ventricles but not in an orderly manner. This is why the heartbeat is irregular and fast.

Clotting and Stroke Risk.

Stroke is the most dangerous and feared complication of a-fib, but it is one that can be managed quite effectively with modern blood thinners. When the atria are fibrillating, the ventricles cannot pump out blood quickly enough, so some of it backs up in the atria. Eventually, if the blood remains there long enough, it can form a clot.

The danger is that this clot can get dislodged and travel to the brain where it may cause a stroke. This sometimes occurs when the heart switches back into normal rhythm and the clot is pushed out into the blood stream. This is why doctors recommend that anyone who has been in a-fib for more than 24-48 hours continuously to take blood thinning medicines or have a scan prior to any treatment to restore a normal heart rhythm.

Your doctor will decide whether or not you need to take blood thinners. The treatment you will receive will depend on how many risk factors you have for stroke. This depends on age, whether or not you have heart disease, diabetes or a prior stroke, your sex and whether or not you have high blood pressure.

Blood thinning medicines can greatly prevent your chances of having an a-fib related stroke. Not everyone will need to take blood thinners, but this must be decided by a qualified health professional. People with lone a-fib and no risk factors have been found in studies to have no higher risk of stroke than other people of the same age who don't have a-fib. However, this is something that needs to be discussed with your health care provider.

Conventional Treatments for Afib

A-fib can present quite a challenge for a doctor. The usual approach is to look for an obvious cause, including heart disease, high blood pressure or thyroid disorders. An echocardiogram which is an ultrasound scan of the heart may be ordered to look for any problems with the structure of the heart or the valves. A blood panel may be requested to check for thyroid and potassium levels.

Unfortunately, for many patients this is where the detective work ends. If no treatable cause can be found, doctors usually prescribe either anti-arrhythmic drugs, drugs to slow the heart down or even refer the patient for an ablation procedure which puts tiny scars around the pulmonary veins in the heart in the hope that it will block the rogue electrical signals which start afib.

Whilst many of these medications work effectively, at least for a time, they are not without side effects. Ironically, most anti-arrhythmic drugs can actually cause arrhythmias, some of which are more serious than those they are trying to prevent! Ablations can be curative at least in the short term (long term data is still lacking due to this being a relatively new procedure) but again are not without risk. Around 1-5% of ablation procedures lead to some sort of complication, most fortunately minor but some extremely serious such as stroke, atrio-oesophageal fistula and even death.

From a patient's perspective, it is certainly sensible to at least look at some natural or alternative treatments which can safely be used alongside conventional medical treatments to manage the condition. The body has a remarkable ability to heal itself when allowed to, and an educated patient and interested physician can make a formidable team when it comes to tacking the condition.

Recognised Causes of A-fib

These are some of the commonest recognised cause of a-fib:

Problems with the structure of the heart, particularly the valves. Mitral valve problems in particular are associated with the occurrence of a-fib.

Hypertension – high blood pressure. Uncontrolled high blood pressure can damage the heart's electrical system.

Heart surgery. - A-fib is a recognised complication of heart surgery. Up to 50% of patients who have cardiac surgery have some degree of post-operative a-fib.

Coronary artery disease – Between 18 and 47% of patients with a-fib have coronary artery disease.

Previous heart attack or damage to the heart from viruses. Anything that damages the electrical system of the heart, from previous heart attack to a virus which attacks the heart muscle can cause a—fib.

Congenital heart defects – 25-30% of patients with congenital heart disease also have a-fib.

Thyroid imbalance – particularly overactive thyroid. Overactive thyroid has such a strong link with atrial fibrillation that doctors routinely test thyroid levels when a patient present in a-fib.

Obesity – Obesity is rapidly becoming one of the leading causes of a-fib. Obesity is thought to affect the hearts electrical system in two ways. Increased weight leads to stretching of the atria which can make them electrically unstable. Also, obesity increases levels of inflammation in the body.

Lung disorders – Pneumonia is a common cause of transient a-fib as are other conditions which affect levels of oxygen in the blood. A-fib is also often initiated around the pulmonary veins which are the veins which carry oxygenated blood back to the heart.

Stimulants – alcohol, caffeine, nicotine, illegal drugs, monosodium glutamate (MSG) overeating (holiday heart). Transient a-fib is so common in emergency rooms during holiday periods it has even earned the nickname holiday heart. Alcohol in particular is a trigger for a-fib.

Mineral deficiencies – especially magnesium and potassium. Deficiencies of these important minerals are potent initiators of all types of arrhythmias. Whilst potassium is routinely measured in lab tests, magnesium deficiency is thought to affect up to 80% of the population and is very hard to measure without expensive tests.

Sleep apnoea – sleep apnoea has a very strong link with a-fib. If you snore or suffer from tiredness in the day time, it may worth getting a sleep study.

Physical and mental stress. In almost every study on a-fib, a large percentage of those questioned said that stress played a role in their attacks. When the body is stressed, chemicals and hormones are released into the blood stream which make the hearts electrical system more excitable.

Viruses – Any virus or indeed anything which puts the body's immune system under strain can trigger a-fib. My first experience with a-fib occurred shortly after a bout of glandular fever.

Diabetes – Diabetes is not only a risk factor for a-fib but increases the risk of stroke and other cardiovascular disease. Inflammation in the body is thought to be one of the reasons that diabetes increases the chance of developing a-fib.

Prescription drug side effects – A-fib can be a side effect of certain drugs, particularly stimulants such as pseudoephedrine, which is often found in decongestant products. Some drugs such as proton pump inhibitors – (omeprazole, Nexium, Prevacid etc.) can lower levels of magnesium if they are taken long term. Magnesium is vital for keeping heart beat regular.

Inflammation – The link between inflammation in the body and a-fib is well established. So much so that some doctors now feel this is the primary mechanism for the development of a-fib. Many of the conditions which are linked to a-fib – obesity, diabetes, sleep apnea, stress are inflammatory conditions. We will talk more in a moment about how inflammation affects the body and how it may trigger a-fib.

Dehydration – Dehydration depletes electrolytes which are essential for maintaining a regular heartbeat. Alcohol leads to dehydration as well as depleting magnesium – a two-pronged attack on the mechanism designed to maintain a regular heartbeat. Athletes and in particular endurance and marathon runners are prone to a-fib which occurs in an otherwise healthy heart. Doctors have speculated whether this is due to long term mineral deficiency or a form of low level dehydration caused by the additional demands on their bodies.

Inflammation and A-fib

Could chronic levels of inflammation in the body contribute to or even cause a—fib? The latest research points to a link, not only between inflammation and a-fib but also many ongoing and chronic diseases. Inflammation is the bodies way of fighting back against injury, toxins and infections. When cells are in distress, they release chemicals which alert the immune system to send help. In return, the immune system sends "fighter cells" to trap the invaders.

When you have a cut or injury you can see the immune system in action. The area may swell, turn red or be warmer than normal. However, this inflammatory response also occurs when internal cells become injured by threats that we cannot see. This may be a sedentary lifestyle, overeating, alcohol, obesity, chronic low grade infections, stress, environmental toxins – the list is endless. Our bodies immune systems end up on a state of high alert and many researchers now believe that is this form of chronic inflammation which sets in motion many types of illness. Inflammation has been linked to heart disease, Alzheimer's, arthritis, depression, asthma, autism, gallbladder disease, multiple sclerosis, stroke – in fact it can affect all systems of the body and manifest all types of disease.

So how does all this tie into a-fib? Levels of inflammation in the body can be measured by a substance called c-reactive protein (CRP) which appears in the blood when there is an inflammatory response in the body. Levels of CRP have been found to be much higher in patients with a-fib than in those with a normal heartbeat. What is more, those in permanent a-fib have higher levels of CRP than those who just have episode of a-fib with normal heart rhythm in between (paroxysmal a-fib). This certainly points to a link between inflammation and a-fib.

Once of the first researchers to study this in depth was Bruins et al in their study "Activation of the complement system during and after cardiopulmonary bypass surgery: post-surgery activation involves C-reactive protein and is associated with postoperative arrhythmia". I have included the full title of the study in case anyone would like to research it further.

In short, the study found that a-fib occurred most often after heart surgery on days 2 and 3. This was when levels of CRP were at their highest, which ties into the body's immune response to the insult of surgery. Further studies have found that giving patients the anti-inflammatory and antioxidant Vitamin C after heart surgery, significantly decreases the chances of patients going into a-fib after the procedure.

It seems then, that there is an indisputable link between a-fib and inflammation. The fact that a-fib frequently occurs with other conditions such as obesity, diabetes and coronary artery disease only serves to further increase inflammation.

Treating A-fib By Reducing Inflammation.

The first step in trying to treat a-fib naturally is to seek to reduce inflammation in the body as much as possible. Whilst the complementary treatments in the chapters that follow may work on their own, they will be most effective when combined with an anti-inflammatory regime.

Diet

A modern diet packed with sugar, salt, processed foods and chemicals produces a sustained inflammatory response in the body. Sugar is one of the worst culprits for causing inflammation. Eating a diet high in sugar has been likened to throwing petrol on a fire. Fibre and the phytonutrients found in fresh fruit, vegetables and nuts on the other hand are anti-inflammatory foods.

Omega 3 is a fatty acid which is found in oily fish, walnuts, flax seed and flax seed oil, canola oil and soybean oil. Studies have found that not only does Omega 3 help to stop inflammation in the body, it can also reverse inflammation that is already present. The jury is still out on whether Omega 3 can benefit a-fib directly, some studies have said it does whilst others have found no effect whatsoever.

Whilst there are numerous books and articles devoted to anti-inflammatory diets, the principle is simple. Avoid processed food, sugars, simple carbs and trans fat. Eat fibre rich natural foods, high amounts of fruit and vegetables, oily fish and nuts. The Paleo diet which is based on our caveman ancestor's diet is considered to be anti-inflammatory although many people find it a little too restrictive for modern living. Nevertheless, some people have reported freedom from atrial fibrillation by following the Paleo Diet or a slightly less restrictive version of it.

Tackle Food Intolerances And Trigger Foods

If you have a food intolerance, it will trigger an inflammatory response every time you eat that food. This reaction is probably best illustrated by celiac disease which is a reaction to the gluten found in wheat, barley and rye. If a person who has gluten intolerance continues to eat food containing gluten, eventually it will seriously damage their intestines.

Lactose intolerance is another common problem, but it is possible to develop a reaction to any food – even healthy foods such as fruit and vegetables. For whatever reason, your body will begin to see that particular food as the enemy so will send out it's army to tackle the offender which leads to the inflammatory response.

If you think a particular food may be causing problems then eliminate it from your diet and see if symptoms improve. Keeping a food diary is a good way of tracking whether certain foods are an issue for you.

Trigger Foods

Trigger foods are foods which have been known to trigger a-fib attacks in susceptible people. Not everyone has the same trigger foods, but the ones described below are common culprits for initiating attacks:

Monosodium Glutamate: MSG

MSG is such a well-known trigger for a-fib attacks that doctors have even coined the term Chinese Restaurant Syndrome to describe attacks which begin after its ingestion. MSG is a common ingredient in Chinese and Asian cooking, although many restaurants are now beginning to omit it.

MSG is also known as E621 and Vetsin and is used as a flavour enhancer in savoury foods. It is found in crisps (chips) and snacks, ready meals, sauces and dressings and in large amounts in some Chinese restaurant meals.

Symptoms of MSG sensitivity usually start within 2 hours of consuming it and can be extremely unpleasant. Symptoms may include arrhythmia and erratic heartbeat, headache, nausea, hot flushes, numbness and burning mouth syndrome.

MSG alone can trigger a-fib as was discovered in a report in the International Journal of Cardiology (Feb 9 2009). The patient was actually a doctor who was considering ablation for his episodic a-fib. After removing MSG and aspartame (another potent trigger) from his diet, his a-fib ceased completely. To prove it had indeed been MSG that had been causing his problems he deliberately ingested it. Within hours his a-fib had returned.

Tyramine
If red wine and aged cheeses trigger your a-fib then your problem could be caused by tyramine. Tyramine is a chemical which occurs naturally in some foods including aged and fermented cheese, fermented foods such as sauerkraut, sour dough, yeast extract, fish, meat, yoghurt, wine, sour cream and over-ripe or dried fruits. Unfortunately for us chocoholics, it is also present in chocolate!

Whilst alcohol alone can be a trigger of a-fib, red wine seems to particularly present a problem for some. This is due to the high levels of tyramine in red wine, which occurs as part of the aging process. Tyramine containing foods should be avoided by patients taking drugs called MAO Inhibitors as they can lead to dangerously high blood pressure.

Aspartame
The artificial sweetener aspartame which is also known as E951, appears in many low calorie, sugar free or low sugar products. It is most commonly used in fizzy drinks but it can

also appear in desserts, shakes, sweeteners and even in some medications, vitamins and toothpaste. 1 in 25 a-fib sufferers studied citied aspartame as being a trigger for attacks.

Alcohol
Heavy alcohol consumption can trigger a-fib even in people with no history of the condition. Binge drinking leads to numerous admissions to the emergency room for a-fib during the holiday season, which is why alcohol induced a-fib is known as holiday heart.

For many people an episode of a-fib caused by overindulgence will be a one-off and so long as they don't drink to excess it may never happen again. For others, even small amounts of alcohol can trigger an attack.

Minerals which help to keep the heart rhythm stable such as magnesium are depleted by alcohol use, and dehydration caused by drinking can reduce levels of these essential minerals even more. If you drink regularly, it is a good idea to keep well hydrated and optimise your mineral levels.

Wheat And Gluten
Research has revealed that the risk of a-fib is slightly higher in people who have gluten sensitivity. Around 1-2% of the population have Celiac Disease (extreme sensitivity to gluten) and 30% of people carry markers for the disease. It is estimated that 80% of celiac patients are undiagnosed.

As with anything which the body is sensitive to, gluten will cause inflammation in susceptible people. Symptoms of celiac disease include diarrhoea, abdominal cramping and pain, bloating, weight loss, lethargy, vomiting, plus seemingly unrelated syndromes such as skin rashes and epilepsy.

Some of us can be sensitive to gluten without developing full blown celiac disease. Celiac disease invokes a response from the immune system and anti-bodies are produced in the blood. Testing for anti-bodies is the first stage in the diagnosis of Celiac Disease and may be followed by a biopsy of the gut. Intolerance on the other hand brings on symptoms which vary with the length and type of exposure.

Some people have reported dramatic improvements in a-fib when switching to a gluten free diet. Of these many have reported an immediate improvement of symptoms but to be completely certain that gluten is the problem it may be necessary to continue the diet for an extended period of time. It may surprise you to learn that gluten can hang around in the body for several months – the half-life of a gluten antibody is around 3-4 months.

Salt

Salt, when eaten in excess can trigger a-fib. When salty foods are eaten the body tries to prevent the ensuing dehydration by retaining fluid. This will in turn raise blood pressure. Salt also depletes the essential healthy heartbeat minerals potassium and magnesium.

In order for the heart's electrical system to function correctly, levels of sodium and potassium are kept strictly in balance. If too much salt is consumed the body releases potassium to counteract this. Whilst most people who eat a normal diet will never become sodium deficient, potassium deficiency can be a trigger and an issue for people with a-fib.

Substituting table salt for one of the potassium chloride based alternatives may help to balance things out but please speak to your doctor first. Potassium can be dangerous for some people, particularly those who have problems with their kidneys.

Whilst salt is essential for maintaining certain functions in the body, almost all of us who eat a Western Diet consume too much of it. In the UK the guidelines are to consume no more than 6g per day. Cutting back on salt will increase the body's ability to retain potassium, which is vital for maintaining a healthy heartbeat.

Dairy Products
In those with true lactose intolerance, eating dairy products containing lactose will trigger an inflammatory response. However, calcium, of which dairy products is an excellent source, is essential to the proper functioning of the heart. Low levels of calcium in the body prolong the QT interval – this is the measurement of the depolarisation and repolarisation of the ventricles. This can lead to dangerous heart rhythms stemming from the bottom of the heart.

Maintaining adequate calcium levels therefore is essential to the function of the heart. Ironically, too much calcium can excite the heart, hence the use of calcium channel blocker drugs in heart disease. If you are worried about too much or too little calcium your doctor will be able to advise you.

Sugar
Since the early 1990's, diabetes has been recognised as an independent risk factor for the development of a-fib. Since then, numerous studies have found that a-fib is linked to high blood sugar. However, what is not so well known is that even in people with normal blood sugar, high sugar consumption increases the risk of heart disease, a-fib and other arrhythmias. Sugar and high glycaemic foods are extremely inflammatory.

Diabetes is an inflammatory condition and diabetics have higher levels of the inflammatory marker c-reactive protein

(CRP) than people with normal blood sugar. A-fib patients also have elevated CRP so a diabetic who also has a-fib is likely to have very high levels of inflammation in the body.

A diet which is high in sugar and high in carbohydrates sets you on the road to diabetes. At first, your body can handle the high levels of sugar in your blood by pumping out insulin which lowers blood sugar. Eventually though, this mechanism starts to fail. Cells start to become resistant to insulin and the pancreas cannot cope with demand. Overall levels of blood sugar start to rise. This doesn't happen overnight but in stages. You may have what is known as impaired fasting glucose – this means that your blood sugar is higher than normal but not high enough to be diabetic, when you haven't eaten for 12 hours or so. Or impaired glucose tolerance – when your blood sugar remains too high 2 hours after you have been given a measured dose of glucose. Eventually, you may go on to develop Type 2 diabetes.

The positive news is that in most cases blood sugars can be normalised, often from just diet alone. Even type 2 diabetics have "reversed" their disease by adopting diets which are low in carbohydrates. A very promising study known as the "Newcastle Study" carried out in the UK found that diabetics of less than 10 years standing could reverse their disease by adopting a very low calorie diet for a period of time or by losing substantial amounts of weight.

Even if you have perfect blood sugar, a high carb high sugar diet puts you at risk of mineral deficiencies – in particular Magnesium. We will talk much more about this essential mineral and how a deficiency can cause a-fib later. If you are still not convinced that sugar is a problem though, consider a report published in the American Journal of Medicine.   In that study, people who got a fifth of their daily calories from sugar (and some of us get a lot more!) increased their risk of dying from heart attack or stroke by 28%.

Resolve Magnesium Deficiency

Magnesium deficiency is very common in the general population with estimates that up to 80% of us have less than optimal levels. If you have diabetes or any form of elevated blood sugar, then you are also certain to be magnesium deficient. One of the manifestations of magnesium deficiency is an erratic heartbeat or a-fib.

It has been known for many years that low levels of minerals will provoke arrhythmia even in healthy hearts. Even short periods of magnesium depletion can bring on heart rhythm changes. One small but really interesting study found that nearly a quarter of women in the study developed a-fib after a relatively short period of magnesium restriction. (Journal of The American College of Nutrition Apr 2007).
Many of us have been deficient in this essential mineral for years!

Since the 1950s the amount of magnesium we naturally get in our diets has dwindled. Levels of magnesium in fruits and vegetables have dropped by 16% and 24% respectively. Processing and cooking food reduces the mineral content further.

Unfortunately there is no accurate or quick way of testing magnesium levels in our bodies unless we resort to very expensive tests. The standard test for magnesium levels is a blood test, but just 1% of the bodies stores of magnesium is contained in the blood. The body actually shifts magnesium out of the major organs in order to maintain levels in the blood. So you can be told you have normal levels from a blood test whereas in fact you actually have a severe deficiency.

Symptoms of a Magnesium Deficiency

Muscle twitching, spasms, tics
Irritability
Anxiety and panic attacks
Tiredness and lethargy
Inability to sleep
Inability to "Switch Off"
Seizures
Irregular or rapid heartbeat
Coronary spasms
Potassium deficiency
Impaired glucose tolerance
Hyperglycaemia
Tremors
Difficulty swallowing
Dizziness
Numbness and tingling
PMS
High blood pressure
Carb cravings
Craving for salt
Insomnia
Loss of appetite
Nausea
GERD
Confusion
Personality changes
Asthma and breathing difficulties
Chronic fatigue syndrome
ADHD
Tooth decay
Gum disease.

Magnesium Deficiency and Atrial Fibrillation

Magnesium plays a major role in the electrical function of the heart. Tissue which does not have adequate magnesium can become electrically unstable leading to arrhythmias and premature beats.

Several researchers have put forward the idea that arrhythmias in structurally normal hearts can be caused by nutritional or mineral deficiency. Dr Matthias Rath has written on the subject quite extensively and his research can be found online.

Athletes are prone to idiopathic arrhythmias and marathon runners and competitive cyclists in particular seem prone to developing "lone" a-fib. It seems a paradox that these athletes who are very physically fit should develop such an ailment. Athletes tend to have very high vagal tone which is another clue to the fact that a-fib could be a disorder of the nervous system. It could be that the enlargement of the heart seen in athletic fitness stretches the atria and makes them more prone to misfire. Or indeed it could be that the very high demands that athletes place on their bodies robs them of essential minerals such as magnesium.

I am one of the many a-fibbers who claim to have cured their a-fib by magnesium repletion alone. You can read my story in the back of the book but co-incidentally in my youth I was an endurance athlete – a competitive swimmer. I consider myself cured so long as I maintain adequate levels of magnesium in my body. If I slack off my regime after a couple of weeks I will start to feel ectopic beats. I read my body for signs of low minerals – eyelid and muscle twitching, skipped beats, or an uneasy panicky feeling and up my intake if necessary. I'm free of a-fib so for me magnesium has been nothing short of a miracle.

Resolving Magnesium Deficiency.

Just as it can take months to years for a mineral deficiency to arise, so it can take months to years to correct it. If you try magnesium for just a short time and decide it doesn't work, it could be that you haven't taking it long enough to correct a deficiency. As ever, I will insert the disclaimer – always consult your physician before adding any vitamin or mineral to your regime. Although magnesium is generally considered safe, it should not be taken by people with certain kidney conditions.

The other problem could be that you are using the wrong type of magnesium. Some forms of magnesium are very poorly absorbed by the body, with as little as 4% of the mineral actually being used. Also it may be ironic, but the lower the magnesium level the harder it becomes to correct with supplementation. Magnesium also needs an adequate supply of potassium in order to be absorbed and vice versa. Potassium supplementation is closely regulated and rightly so as it can be dangerous if taken without medical supervision. Potassium levels can be accurately measured by blood test so if you think you are low ask your doctor for a test.

Magnesium Rich Foods
The following foods are good natural sources of magnesium and should be incorporated into your diet as much possible.

Pumpkin Seeds
Spinach
Swiss Chard
Yoghurt/Kefir

Almonds
Black Beans
Avocado
Figs
Dark Chocolate
Banana
Salmon
Nuts and Seeds
Coriander
Coffee (in moderation!)
Kelp
Rice Bran

Magnesium Supplementation

Even with the healthiest diet, it can sometimes be difficult to get enough magnesium – particularly if you have extra need for it. Magnesium oxide is the cheapest form of magnesium but is very badly absorbed by the body, just 1/25 of each dose is actually utilised by the body.

More absorbable forms of magnesium include magnesium glycinate, magnesium taurate and magnesium citrate.

Magnesium glycinate is a chelated form of magnesium, which means it is bound to an amino acid which helps it be absorbed into the body. Magnesium glycinate is also less likely to cause loose stools than other forms of magnesium. Approximately 80% of magnesium glycinate is absorbed.

Magnesium taurate is a compound of magnesium and taurine which is an amino acid. Taurine possesses anti-arrhythmic properties, decreases irritability of heart tissues and helps to regulate magnesium, sodium and potassium levels within cells. It is considered a helpful supplement by many people with a-fib and is sometimes used together with arginine to reduce the frequency of ectopic beats – both PVC's and PAC's.

Magnesium citrate is a readily available, cheap and well absorbed form of magnesium but unfortunately it does have laxative effects in higher doses. Magnesium citrate is available in powder form as well as capsules so you can experiment with a dose which doesn't cause bowel problems. Magnesium citrate is excreted quite quickly by your body so it is recommended it is used several times per day in small doses.

Magnesium malate is a form of magnesium which is found helpful by a-fibbers and sufferers of fibromyalgia and chronic fatigue syndrome alike. Malic acid helps to increase energy production and some studies have found it useful in reducing blood pressure although there is not yet enough evidence to consider using it for this purpose alone.

All forms of oral magnesium can have a laxative effect, some more than others. Diarrhoea can worsen a deficiency as the body loses not only magnesium but also potassium and sodium. If you experience loose bowels cut back on oral magnesium and consider using transdermal magnesium which is another highly bio-available form of magnesium.

Transdermal Magnesium

Transdermal magnesium is applied to the skin and is easily absorbed. It is also highly effective in treating muscle aches and pains and sports injuries as well as replenishing stores in the body. Magnesium "oil" is a form of transdermal magnesium which isn't really an oil, but a solution of magnesium chloride in purified water. Other transdermal magnesium products include lotions, gels, foot soaks and bath flakes.

.

Transdermal magnesium can replete body stores approximately five times faster than oral supplementation and has none of the laxative side effects. Magnesium chloride flakes can be added to baths or used as a foot-bath. For a bath dissolve around 250mg (UK measure) of flakes in a bath of warm water and soak for around 20 minutes. In a foot-bath use around 150mg. Repeat 2-3 times per week for optimal efficiency.

Whilst magnesium oils are not expensive, beware of very cheap magnesium products which may be magnesium sulphate (Epsom Salts).   These are not nearly as effective as the standard 31% Zechstein magnesium oils so provide false economy.

Correcting a minor magnesium deficiency with transdermal magnesium takes around 4 – 6 weeks. Oral supplementation takes an average 6 months to achieve the same effect. Side effects are rare but magnesium oil may cause tingling and local irritation on application to start with, particularly if magnesium stores are very low. It is not recommended that you use the product on broken skin but if you do then you may need to dilute the solution to 4% or less.

Magnesium Overdose

Magnesium overdose is very rare in people with normal kidney function as healthy kidneys will filter out the excess. Nevertheless, magnesium overdose could be an issue with renal impairment or when mega amounts of the mineral are ingested.   This is why it is important to check that it is safe to take magnesium with your health care provider prior to supplementation.

Signs of a Magnesium overdose
Low blood pressure
Slow breathing
Slow heart rate and or erratic heart rhythm
Shortness of breath
Dizziness
In very severe cases cardiac arrest

If you or someone else has consumed very large doses of magnesium and the above signs appear seek immediate medical care.

Treat low level infection.

Low level chronic infection in the body taxes the immune system and increases levels of inflammation. If your body is constantly keeping minor infections in check it cannot work as hard when a crisis occurs. Consider an army who has deployed a quarter of its troops into far flung corners of the world. If a war starts, it would be left seriously disadvantaged.

So what do we mean by low level chronic infection? Gum disease is one example. Nearly half of all adults have some form of gum disease, and it can put you at much greater risk of heart attack or stroke. Once in the blood stream, bacteria from teeth and gums can travel directly to the heart. In rare cases the bacteria can damage a heart valve – a condition known as endocarditis.

H-Pylori

Another form of low level infection is caused by bacteria which live in the stomach of over 50% of the world's population. These bacteria are known as h-pylori and for many people they don't cause a problem. However, in others h-pylori causes a chronic inflammation of the stomach leading to gastritis and ulcers. Over 90% of stomach ulcers are believed to be caused by h-pylori.

A-fib patients are 20 times more likely to test positive for h-pylori than healthy volunteers. Not only that by their levels of the inflammatory marker – CRP were five times as high. If this does not convince you that a-fib and inflammation are linked, then nothing will!

Eradication of h-pylori has eliminated a-fib in some patients. Unfortunately, the bug is a tough little critter designed to survive in even the harshest conditions in the stomach. It burrows into the walls of the gut and protects itself in a layer of ammonia. In many people this causes no symptoms at all, others will develop upper abdominal pain, nausea, vomiting or even an ulcer. Unless h-pylori is eliminated effectively from the body, it can remain there indefinitely.

Any person who has a-fib should be tested for h-pylori. There are three main ways of testing – blood, breath or stool tests. Your doctor will advise on which one is most suitable for you.

Eradicating H-Pylori

The most common way of eradicating h-pylori is with a combination of drugs known as triple therapy. Usually this is two different anti-biotics and a proton pump inhibitor which reduces levels of stomach acid. This is successful around 85% of the time. If it fails, it is usually repeated with a different combination of drugs.

A natural treatment for h-pylori is Mastic Gum. This is a gum made from the resin of a tree native to Greece. It has been used for centuries for stomach problems, but recently it has been found to supress and even kill h-pylori.

Whilst Mastic is not as effective as anti-biotics for clearing up the bacteria, it nevertheless has some potential. One study (1) [i] found that Mastic gum alone eradicated h-pylori in 30% and 38% of the groups studied in just 14 days. Mastic has low toxicity and few side effects.

Other low level infections include bacterial vaginosis, chronic ear infections, sinus problems, Lyme disease and skin infections. By choosing to get these actively treated, you will reduce inflammation in your body.

Don't Be Sedentary

Living a sedentary lifestyle increases markers for inflammation in the blood. Exercise has been shown to reduce these bio-markers as well as improving many other aspects of health. Just three hours of exercise per week – or half an hour every day can cut your risk of heart attack in half!

On the other hand, excessive exercise can also contribute to a-fib. It is a well-known but puzzling fact that many marathon runners, endurance athletes, cyclists and swimmers develop the condition. Most a-fib in athletes is classed as lone a-fib as these highly fit individuals rarely have any underlying heart conditions. A disorder of the vagal nervous system, dehydration, mineral deficiencies or occult damage to the heart's electrical system through over-training have all been put forward as possible theories as to why this happens.

Before beginning any exercise regime, it is important to get your doctors consent. In order to be beneficial, exercise does not have to be extreme. Even gentle exercise taken regularly has a positive effect on the body.

Treat Sleep Apnea

Sleep apnea is a condition where you stop breathing in your sleep, often many times a night. Consequently, sleep is disturbed and sufferers experience daytime sleepiness and fatigue. You may have no recollection of this when you wake-up, and it is often noticed by a partner. Signs of sleep apnea include loud snoring, snorting, gasping and choking. If you suspect you may have the condition, an overnight sleep study in a special laboratory can confirm it.

The link between sleep apnea and a-fib is so strong that some researchers now believe that sleep apnea actually causes a-fib rather than being a co-existing condition. Untreated sleep apnea can stop anti-arrhythmic drugs from working properly and it also increases the chance of a-fib recurring after a cardioversion (an electric shock designed to make your heart return to a normal rhythm) or an ablation.

The prevalence of sleep apnea in people with a-fib is actually quite astonishing. Studies have revealed that at least 40% and perhaps up to 80% of people with a-fib have obstructive sleep apnea. In one study (*Bitter T, Langer C, Vogt J, Horstkotte D, Oldenburg O 2009*) OSA was found in 42.7% of patients with a-fib. In another even more shocking study (*Braga B, Poyares D, Cintra F et al 2009*) the number was found to be 81.6%!

In the general population, sleep apnea affects 5-10% of adults. A-fibbers therefore, are up to 16 times more likely to have the condition. The relationship has also been found to be true in reverse. Someone who has sleep apnea but no a-fib has a four times increased chance of developing the condition in the future.

The risk of developing sleep apnea is increased if you are overweight and as body mass rises, the risk increases even more. It is interesting that obstructive sleep apnea (OSA) alone can cause weight gain and if the condition is controlled, it can be much easier to lose weight.

Left untreated, OSA can be quite serious, but it is relatively easy to treat using a CPAP device. CPAP stands for continuous positive airway pressure and takes the form of a mask which is worn during sleep which uses air pressure to hold the airway open. Alternatively, if your apnea is mild, your doctor may recommend lifestyle changes such as weight loss or stopping smoking to see if it improves.

If you have a-fib it is certainly worth speaking to your medical practitioners about your risk of sleep apnea and following their advice. CPAP has been found to reduce the risk of recurrence by up to 42%.

Weight Loss and Afib

For a long time, doctors have thought that being overweight contributes to the development of a-fib. Just recently though, several studies have released that losing weight not only reduces inflammation in the body, but significantly reduces or even reverses a-fib.

In one very positive study, researchers found that nearly half of those studied achieved a total remission of symptoms if they lost just 10% of their body weight.

In a presentation at the American College of Cardiology's 64th Annual Scientific Session, the researchers concluded that patients who lost 10% of their body weight were six times more likely to achieve freedom from a-fib than those who failed to lose weight.

It was also found that sustained weight loss was an important factor in remaining a-fib free. Those patients who regained weight or their weight fluctuated by 5% or more weren't as successful in maintaining a steady heartbeat.

Obesity affects the heart in many ways. It puts the heart under extra strain increasing the chance of high blood pressure, increases inflammation in the blood vessels and in some cases can even make the heart increase in size. This stretches the top part of the heart (the atria) leading to an increased risk of disordered electrical signals.   It is these errant signals that can trigger a-fib, particularly when they start around the pulmonary veins.

It is not just the top part of the heart that is affected by obesity. The bottom chambers of the heart – the ventricles are responsible for the bulk of the pumping action of the heart. Obesity can damage their structure and function which can lead to heart failure or arrhythmia.

The chance of developing a-fib rises as body mass index (BMI) increases. The risk of developing afib increases by up to 5% for every point that BMI rises.   Obese people tend to have larger atria than non-obese people, which leads to increased atrial pressure, stretch and slower and more disordered conduction of electrical signals.

Obese people also have shorter atrial refractory periods (the resting period of the atria) than people of normal weight. During refractory periods a-fib cannot be initiated. This makes the hearts of obese patients more prone to going into a-fib due to the shorter rest period. If you overload a car, you increase the chance of the engine misfiring.

Whilst it has been established for many years that obesity contributes to a-fib, it is only recently that it has been definitely proven that weight loss improves and even reverses a-fib.

The first long term study to look at how sustained weight loss affects afib was published in 2015, by R Pathak, a cardiologist and fellow of electrophysiology at the University of Adelaide. 355 participants were enrolled in the study which took place over four years.

At the end of the study, 45% of patients who lost over 10% of their body weight remained free from afib symptoms without the use of medication or surgery. 22% of patients who lost between 3 and 9% of their body weight also remained free of symptoms. The weight loss also beneficially impacted the structure of the heart, plus a number of other factors including blood pressure, blood sugar and lipids. The results proved that weight loss could be as beneficial as certain anti-arrhythmic drugs.

Losing weight can even help if you have scheduled an ablation for your a-fib. It can improve surgical access and make the experience easier and less risky. An Australian study found that patients who lost weight, had a five times higher chance of having a successful ablation and remaining in normal rhythm than patients who did not.

An Ideal Diet for A-Fib?

According to studies, sustained gradual weight loss is very effective so a generally heart-healthy diet coupled with moderate exercise is ideal for most people. In the study looking at the effect weight loss had on ablation outcomes *(R Pathak et al: Dec 2014)* patients were initially fed a high protein, low GI calorie controlled diet. If, after 3 months the participants had failed to lose 3% or more of their body weight, very low calories meal replacements were substituted for 1 or 2 meals per day. Participants also started with 20 minutes 3 times per week of low intensity exercise increasing to 200 minutes of moderate intensity exercise a week.

Whilst no a-fib specific diet has yet been developed, anecdotal evidence from a-fibbers have found some things to be beneficial. The most obvious is to avoid potential triggers such as alcohol, refined sugars, food additives such as MSG and gluten if you are sensitive. Optimise your intake of the a-fibbers favourite minerals such as potassium and magnesium, lower your intake of salt and moderate your intake of the cardiac excitatory calcium.

Other a-fibbers have reported vast improvements and even total freedom from afib with the Paleo diet and other forms of low carbohydrate diet such as the Atkins. As a complete carboholic, I have great difficult in staying away from bread and other yummy carbs for long periods, although when I was an a-fibber, several of my episodes began shortly after a high carb meal.

Nevertheless, as the study revealed, the key to success is being able to sustain the weight loss and maintain your weight within a 5% margin, so it is important to find a diet which is sensible and that you can stick to, crash diets or very restrictive menu plans are unlikely to set you up for long term success.

Like all forms of alternate therapies, it is important to work with your doctor before embarking on a new diet or exercise plan. This is particularly important if you are taking blood thinners such as Warfarin which may interact with some food stuffs particularly those containing Vitamin K. Losing weight can also significantly reduce blood sugar, so if you are diabetic this may mean that your doctor needs to reduce your medication. Also, if you have kidney problems, minerals such as potassium, salt and fluids may need to be restricted.

Of course, not everyone who has atrial fibrillation is overweight, and there are some a-fibbers who have the physique of a racing snake. But, if you are overweight and have afib, shaking those extra pounds may be all you have to do to stay in rhythm.

Reduce Stress

Stress has been known to have an adverse effect on heart rhythm even in the healthiest of hearts. Many people suffer from what they describe as "skipped beats" or the sensation that the heart is missing beats.

In actual fact, what they are describing is not a missed heartbeat at all but an early heartbeat. When the heartbeat is initiated earlier than normal, there is a slightly longer pause whilst the heart fills up with blood ready for the next heartbeat. This pause is often perceived as a missed or skipped heartbeat.

Depending on which part of the heart they occur in, doctors refer to these early beats as PAC's (premature atrial contractions) or PVC's (premature ventricle contractions). They are also known as ectopic beats or palpitations. In the vast majority of cases, they are totally benign and in fact just about all of us suffer from them daily. Most of us don't feel them but for some people, the unpleasant sensation can cause significant anxiety.

As with anything heart-related, always check with your doctor if you are experiencing skipped beats or if your skipped beats significantly increase in number. However, the odds are that he or she will be able to reassure you that nothing sinister is going on.

Stress is a well-known culprit for ectopic beats, but they can also be caused by caffeine, nicotine and tiredness. They may also occur when the vagal nerve – a long nerve which starts in the brain and passes through the neck into the abdomen, becomes irritated. The heart is closely linked to the vagal nerve, and anything which irritates this nerve can also cause palpitations.

Many a-fibbers have linked their episodes to stomach disturbances – particularly when there is a lot of gas in the stomach. In fact, it is the pressure on the vagal nerve which is often the culprit. Patients have told their doctors "I burped and my heart went back into rhythm", the release of gas reduced the pressure on the vagal nerve.

Not so long ago, doctors divided atrial fibrillation into two varieties – "adrenergic" and "vagal". These terms are not so common now, as it is recognised that many a-fibbers do not fall neatly into either category. Adrenergic a-fib was thought to be caused by an imbalance in the sympathetic nervous system – that which is responsible for the "fight or flight response". Thus adrenergic a-fibbers were sensitive to adrenaline, exercise, stress and exertion. Their attacks seemed to happen mainly in the daytime – particularly the morning, when sympathetic nervous system activity was at its highest.

Vagal a-fibbers on the other hand seemed to experience attacks mainly in the evening, particularly after a main meal or when they were at rest. The vagal nerve is responsible for parasympathetic nervous system activity which slows the heart and calms down the body. If episodes of a-fib occur after eating or right when you are trying to drift off to sleep at night, then it could be the vagal nerve.

Quite why the vagal nerve becomes irritable in some people is not fully understood. However, many potential theories have been put forward from obesity putting pressure on the nerve through to mineral deficiencies in potassium and magnesium making it "cranky". The fact that a-fib episodes improve or even disappear after weight loss or mineral supplementation does add weight to these theories.

One other potential theory and one I personally favour is that high levels of c-reactive protein (the inflammatory marker we discussed earlier) caused by chronic stress, throws the whole body out of whack – including and especially the vagal nerve.

Modern living alone creates chronic low levels of stress in many individuals. Money worries, financial problems, health issues and world events all contribute to "stress" chemicals circulating in our bodies. Doctors often tell us to "reduce stress" but they rarely go into detail about how we are supposed to achieve that. The old advice such as work less or take up a hobby just doesn't cut it in the modern world!

What many doctors fail to understand is that a-fib is a tremendously stressful condition to live with every day. Not only for sufferers but also family members and loved ones. A-fib can have a huge impact on everyday life, due to its unpredictable nature. When I was first diagnosed I was told "It isn't life threatening, so just get on with it". Undoubtedly some people can do that, but I wasn't one of them. I wanted more answers than the doctors could give me, so I researched my condition obsessively. Luckily it was this research which led eventually to my cure.

Educating yourself about a-fib is probably the best thing you can do to reduce stress. Hopefully this book will have provided you with many of the answers you need. By understanding the condition, you are empowering yourself to make educated decisions about your treatment. You will also lose much of the fear when you realise that this is a treatable and often curable condition.

In the next section, we look at some alternative ways of helping a-fib. Many of the suggestions will also be useful for reducing stress.

Acupuncture/Acupressure

Acupuncture has long been considered an effective treatment for palpitations and high blood pressure, but two exciting studies have proved that it is effective as a treatment for a-fib. As we discussed in the chapter on stress, a-fib can be considered as a disorder of the nervous system as well as the heart. Acupuncture is traditionally though to balance the autonomic nervous system by enhancing the flow of energy through the body by puncturing specific areas with needles.

Practitioners of Traditional Chinese Medicine (TCM) have traditionally used the Neiguan (PC-6) acupuncture point to treat heart related conditions. Neiguan is often described as a balancing point - it can help with sickness and nausea, palpitations and to restore nervous system balance.

The Shenmen point (HT-7 or the Spirit Gate) is a calming point and is useful for palpitations, restoring a regular heartbeat and treating anxiety. It has also been used to treat cardiac pain, manic depression and insomnia.

Finally, the Xinshu spot (BL-15) is found to have a calming and balancing effect on the nervous system.

Two major studies have been carried out into how helpful acupuncture can be when treating a-fib and the results were very promising.

In the first study[ii], researchers looked at how effective acupuncture was in preventing a-fib after a cardioversion (treatment to restore a regular heartbeat). Whilst this was a relatively small study (80 patients) the researchers found that acupuncture was almost as effective as the drug amiodarone in preventing recurrences of a-fib.

In a second study[iii], researchers looked at the use of acupuncture as an alternative to drugs when treating persistent and episodic a-fib. Patients were selected to undergo a 10-week course of acupuncture with sessions once a week, puncturing the Neiguan, Shenmen and Xinshu points described above.

The results showed that acupuncture did have a measurable anti-arrhythmic effect for patients with all types of a-fib. For a small group of patients with paroxysmal (episodic) a-fib, acupuncture was extremely effective and significantly reduced both the duration and the frequency of their episodes.

Unfortunately, if you are taking anti-coagulant drugs you may not be able to have acupuncture due to the risk of bleeding. Talk to your medical practitioner.

Whilst acupuncture is generally considered safe in the hands of a qualified and experienced practitioner, it is not for everyone. If you have a metal allergy, infection or certain underlying medical conditions then you may not be suitable for treatment. And obviously if you have a needle phobia then acupuncture is not a good idea!

 A professional acupuncturist will take a full medical history and advise you of any potential problems before you begin. If you are not suitable for acupuncture, then you might want to investigate noninvasive treatments such as acupressure. Acupressure uses the same network of points and meridians but stimulates them with pressure rather than needles.

Yoga

Yoga has been found to be beneficial to many types of irregular heartbeat, including a-fib. Regular practice of yoga can relieve stress, lower blood pressure, balance the nervous system and helps to steady and regulate the heart. A-fib patients who practised yoga regularly were found to have lower resting heart rates and lower blood pressure than those who did not.

Doctor Dhanunjaya Lakkireddy of the University of Kansas Hospital is currently studying the effect of yoga on atrial fibrillation. He believes there is a significant connection between the heart and the brain and that a-fib is critically dependant on communication between the two. This ties in with the modern thinking that a-fib is not just a cardiac disorder but a sign of an imbalance in the body or the nervous system.

When patients participated in hour long yoga sessions, twice a week for three months, they were found to have less episodes of a-fib, lower blood pressure, better general health and a more positive outlook on life. Whilst Dr Lakkireddy stresses that yoga should not be substituted for medical treatment, it can be very helpful as an additional treatment with the permission of your doctor.

Yoga is suitable for almost everyone and can be tailored to any level of fitness or suppleness. Certain types of yoga such as hot yoga may not be suitable for a-fib patients and poses such as The Downward Dog may not be suitable for people with high blood pressure. For this reason, whilst it is possible to learn yoga at home from books, videos and courses, if you have a medical condition it is worthwhile seeking out a professional yoga teacher or local class. This way you can be sure that the exercises are suitable for you and won't damage your health.

The following breathing exercise are adapted from yoga and are very effective. Do not practice them if you have breathing disorders, are pregnant or have uncontrolled high blood pressure.

Energy Breath (Bellows Breath/Stimulating Breath)

Suitable for: Restoring energy, Invigoration

Keeping your mouth closed, breath in and out very quickly – aim for three cycles per second for 10-15 seconds. Breath normally after each cycle. You can gradually increase the amount of time you practice for 5 seconds a time, up to one full minute. Ensure that you breathe normally for at least a minute between each cycle.

Relaxing Breath

Suitable for: Relaxation, Calming the Nervous System

Place the tip of your tongue behind your top front teeth. Purse your lips slightly. Your tongue should stay in this position throughout the entire breathing exercise. Exhale fully through your mouth making a whooshing sound. Close your mouth and breath in through your nose to the count of 4. Hold your breath to the count of 7. Finally exhale through your mouth to the count of 8. This circular breathing motion helps to calm the nervous system and may be useful if you experience ectopic beats when your vagal nerve becomes irritable.

Start with four breath cycles the first time you do it and build up to 8 cycles over time.

Chiropractic Adjustment

Several a-fib patients have reported improvement or even total resolution of symptoms with chiropractic adjustment. A report in the Journal of Upper Cervical Chiropractic Research (Feb 22 2012) documented the story of a lady with daily attacks of atrial fibrillation coupled with high blood pressure whose symptoms resolved after two chiropractic adjustments. Unfortunately, no follow up information is given on the long term success of this method or whether she needed any further treatment.

Chiropractic adjustment dates back over 100 years when Daniel Palmer, a healer from Iowa found that misaligned vertebrae in our spines could significantly impact health. He believed that misaligned vertebrae cause the nervous system to malfunction, resulting in a myriad of different symptoms in many parts of the body.

These symptoms range from neck and back pain, through to more subtle problems such as lack of energy, problems with the digestive system, impaired immune health and cardiovascular symptoms. Spinal misalignment increases sympathetic overdrive (the "revving up" of the nervous system) which is linked to palpitations and atrial fibrillation. In addition, misaligned vertebrae can irritate the vagal nerve which may explain some cases of "vagal a-fib".

If no obvious cardiac cause for a-fib can be established, as is the case with many athletes and "lone" a-fibbers, it may well be worth considering a spinal evaluation with a qualified chiropractor.

Vertebrae can become misaligned for many reasons, in some cases even dating back to birth. It's not just physical trauma that causes misalignment, nutritional deficiencies and even emotional stress can cause it too. Even a slight misalignment in the vertebrae can throw the nervous system out of balance.

Dr Martin Gallagher, a medical doctor and chiropractor, described a young female patient who came to him with palpitations trigged by leaning forward. She found that leaning back would cause the palpitations and chest pressure she was experiencing to cease. Dr Gallagher found that she had a misalignment in the upper part of her thoracic spine. After several adjustments her problem completely resolved.

Misaligned vertebrae have been associated with a host of seemingly unrelated medical conditions including:

Headaches
Vision problems including blurred vision

Tinnitus
Non cardiac chest pain
High Blood Pressure
Digestive Problems
Irritable Bowel Syndrome
Tiredness and Fatigue
Difficulty concentrating
Arthritis and Joint Pain
Chronic viral infections and impaired immune system
Arrhythmia and tachycardia
Palpitations

High blood pressure is a condition which commonly accompanies a-fib and surprisingly this too can be caused by a misalignment of the atlas vertebrae in the top of the spinal column. This can cause an altered blood flow to the brain and also send the nervous system into overdrive which can increase blood pressure.

Unfortunately, there have never been any official studies done into chiropractic adjustment and atrial fibrillation, which may be due to the medical professions reluctance to embrace the practice. Nevertheless, there is a fair amount of anecdotal evidence with patients claiming that it has helped or even cured their a-fib. If you have a-fib which has no apparent cause, and particularly if you have ever had any trauma to your back or neck then chiropractic adjustment may be of interest to you.

As with any form of alternative remedy always check with your doctor and consider the pros and cons. Serious complications are rare in the hands of a fully qualified and experienced practitioner but they can include herniated discs and exacerbation of existing disc problems. Very rarely indeed, neck manipulation may lead to stroke.

Some health insurance policies do cover the costs of chiropractic adjustment, although this might limit your choice of practitioner.

EFT Emotional Freedom Technique

EFT or emotional freedom technique is sometimes referred to as "tapping". It draws from various aspects of alternative medicine including acupuncture and energy therapy. I first heard about EFT when it was reported that a patient had achieved a complete resolution of their symptoms through the technique. [iv] Since then, several a-fib patients have reported full or partial success with the system, which can be easily learned in around 10 minutes.

EFT involves tapping on certain parts of the body whilst repeating phrases or affirmations. The nine points which are tapped are believed to be energy meridians through which the life force of "chi" flows within the body.

The technique has been around since the early 1990's and has been embraced by many alternative health practitioners and metaphysical teachers. Nevertheless, it has attracted its fair share of critics who believe that it is based on "pseudoscience", "quackery" or relies on the placebo effect.

However, some critical studies have recently validated the technique, particularly a report published in the APA journal Review of General Psychology which found that the benefits of EFT provided positive statistical results which far outweighed those which could be expected by chance. Other studies have found that just one session of EFT can reduce traumatic memories and reduce depression.

Basic EFT technique.

There are many books, articles and videos online which go into this technique in much more detail including detailed illustrations of the meridian points. However, I have attempted to outline the basic technique below.

Locating the Tapping Points

1. The Top of the Head – the centre of the top of the head. Imagine you were to draw a line to dissect the top of your head into four quarters. The tapping point is where the lines would meet in the middle.
2. The Edge of the Eyebrow – At start of your eyebrow on the same side as your nose.
3. The Side of the Eye – On the bony point at the side of the eye closest to the ear.
4. Underneath The Eye – On the bony point around 2.5cm from your pupil underneath the eye.
5. Under The Nose – On the midline between the bottom of your nose and the start of the upper lip.
6. Chin – midway between the bottom lip and the point of the chin. Note that this is not actually on the point of the chin
7. Collarbone – This can be a tricky one to find as it is not actually on the collar bone but where the collarbone starts. Find the notch at the top of the breastbone and then move down and across one inch. The notch of the breastbone is around where a man would have the knot of his tie.
8. On the side of the body around 10cm below the armpit.
9. Side of hand. On the outside edge of the hand midway between the wrist and the bottom of the little finger. This is sometimes called the karate chop point.

The tapping technique is done with at least two fingers tapping firmly on each point around five times. You can tap on either side of the body, using whichever hand you like. You can also swap sides if you wish for convenience.

Some practitioners like to start with the point on the side of the hand and then work from the top to the bottom of the body whilst others like to start at the top of the head and work down.

As you tap each point repeat out loud an affirmation which promotes healing or acceptance. Some practitioners of EFT choose not to use "positive" or healing affirmations but instead choose to focus on reality and acceptance. The idea behind this is not to change things but to accept and is based on the belief that physical symptoms are a manifestation of emotional "scars or trauma" and only by accepting them can we move on and overcome them.

This esoteric way of thinking may be a leap too far for many of us so one way of overcoming the problem is the "acceptance/choice" technique. For a-fib an example might be – "Even though I have atrial fibrillation (acceptance) I choose to have a steady regular heartbeat (choice). Or "Even though I have an irregular heartbeat I choose to have a healthy heart".

The EFT technique can and has been applied to many aspects of life – from overcoming the scars of trauma and abuse, through to dealing with the symptoms of physical illness. It may help to ease some of the anxiety and fear which often accompanies a-fib.

Toward A More Positive Future

I hope that the strategies and information in this book have been helpful to you. Knowledge is your greatest ally in dealing with this condition. Being an informed patient will help you and your doctors to make the best decisions about your health.

Whichever route you decide to take on your a-fib journey, whether it be conventional medical treatment or a combination of natural and medical treatment under the guidance of your doctors, it is reassuring to know that great advances have been made in the treatment of this condition. Barely twenty year ago the only medical treatments were either anti-arrhythmic drugs or an open heart surgical treatment known as The Maze. Blood thinning usually required patients to take Warfarin or for those at lower risk of clots, Aspirin.

We now have a range of new blood thinners which do not require such stringent monitoring, plus ablation techniques which give patients a real hope for a permanent cure. However perhaps most exciting, is the research which links a-fib with modifiable risk factors such as obesity, diet and stress. A-fib is no longer seen as purely a heart condition, other factors such as imbalances of the nervous system, inflammation in the body and nutritional deficiencies are increasingly being recognised as potential causes.

Working with a qualified medical practitioner who is also open to natural treatments and the impact of lifestyle changes is invaluable. I have stressed throughout this book that you should always take the advice of your medical practitioner before adopting any of the strategies herein. However, that also requires a doctor who is willing to take a holistic approach to the condition. There is no "one size fits all" approach with a-fib. It is a condition which can pose a great challenge to the diagnostician. If you have been told you have "lone" a-fib which occurs for no particular reason, as I was, you and your doctor have a great deal of detective work ahead of you. If there is nothing structurally wrong with your heart, then it may be an imbalance of the nervous system, the gastric system, chronic inflammation or even a food intolerance that may be causing your problem.

A-fib is often described by doctors as none life threatening but what many forget is that it can be incredibly life changing. Some patients leave the hospital with a new diagnosis of a-fib filled with anxiety and fear for the future. They may not fully understand the diagnosis and this can lead to extreme anxiety and depression. Yet a-fib is a condition which can be managed effectively and no-one should live in fear. New treatments, approaches and research into the condition offer hope for the future. Even in permanent a-fib it is possible to live a long and productive life and hundreds of thousands of people all over the world are proving that every day.

I wish you every success on your journey to beat a-fib. The very best of health to you.

My A-Fib Story and How I Cured Myself

I included this story in my first book on a-fib "Conquer Your Afib" so apologies to those who are already familiar with it.

My first experience with a-fib occurred in the summer of 2001. Like most 31-year-old females, prior to this I never gave my heartbeat a second thought, I was busy finishing my degree as a mature student and life was hectic.

The simple act of the mail arriving changed my life forever. My dog barked and startled me and as I bent over to pick up the mail I felt my heart take off in a crazy rhythm. It felt like it was beating at around 100mph, it was flip flopping all over the place, skipping beats and it felt like it was trying to jump out of my chest. I was gripped with panic as I began to feel light headed and dizzy, I was thinking "Is this a heart attack? A stroke? It felt like something was very wrong but I did not know what.

For reasons which I still can't explain, rather than going straight to accident and emergency, I sought an emergency appointment with my GP. An hour later I was sat in her office, my heart was still beating wildly and crazily out of control, I was panicking and now I also had an intense desire to rush to the toilet every few minutes.

An ECG revealed that my heart was indeed racing at around 150 beat per minute and the problem was occurring in the top part of my heart rather than the bottom. That means it is not life threatening said my doctor although at that point I was far from reassured!

I was sent to the hospital in a taxi as it had been decided it wasn't urgent enough to call an ambulance and I certainly wasn't allowed to drive myself. My diagnosis was either supraventricular tachycardia, atrial fibrillation or atrial flutter. About half way to the hospital I felt my heart rhythm change, it started to feel regular and was slowing down. An ECG at the hospital revealed that my heart was indeed beating normally again although it was still a little fast at 110-120bpm – no doubt due to my state of anxiety.

Unfortunately, the hospital had lost my original ECG print out from my doctors but more than made up for it by keeping me in for three days for tests. At the end of it and after a complete barrage of tests all we had was a list of conditions I definitely did not have and nothing conclusive to explain what I did have. My heart was structurally perfect, my heart function as great, I had not had a heart attack, all blood results were normal, ECG was fine and my thyroid was fine.

Three days later, a doctor came and sat beside my bed. "We think we know what you have" she said. "Don't worry, it is not life threatening and we can control it". She went on to explain how they thought I had a condition called paroxysmal atrial fibrillation. Whilst it is often connected to heart problems, in some people without underlying cardiac disease it "just happened". Unfortunately, I was one of those people. I had lone a-fib and no-one had any answers. What I did learn was that a-fib was uncommon in younger people and even less common in women. "Why me?" was my immediate question. "We just don't know" said the doctors. I was told to go away, life my life and stop worrying. "A-fib won't kill you", said the doctors. "In fact you have much the same life expectancy as the general population".

Not worrying is not something I am particularly good at, and when I got home I consulted Dr Google. That was a mistake. Up until that time, no-one had mentioned that I could be at risk of stroke or heart failure. In fact, no-one had mentioned that a-fib was particularly serious at all. In 2001, the main hope for a cure lay with the Maze procedure which involved open heart surgery or an experimental ablation technique which was very much in its infancy. Everything I read on a-fib was scary, and predicted that within 15 years my atrial fibrillation would have progressed from paroxysmal to permanent. Everything seemed to be doom and gloom

In the years that followed I had several more a-fib attacks some lasting seconds and some lasting over 9 hours. Every day I would get flutters and skipped beats and when the" big attacks" hit I would lie still in my bed frightened to move for hours. I suffered from extreme anxiety even when I wasn't in a-fib. I wouldn't make plans for fear I would have an attack, I avoided driving and I seemed to live constantly with my finger hovering over my pulse checking whether or not I was in a regular rhythm.

I also began to read just about everything I could on a-fib trying to find the answers that the doctors just couldn't give me. Eventually I came across an article by Dr Carolyn Dean about the symptoms of magnesium deficiency. Whilst I had just about every symptom on the list the one that stood out for me was the irregular heartbeat. A-fib can occur in a structurally normal heart when there is a deficiency of magnesium. The next article I read was a lady who had cured her irregular heartbeat completely with magnesium alone.

Years of a very bad diet, stress and an eating disorder had eroded my magnesium stores to virtually nothing. I immediately went out and purchased magnesium supplements, I had no clue which type I was buying or that certain types of magnesium are more effective than others. By chance I purchased the chelated type. Within hours, the skips and missed heartbeats were significantly decreased. Within days they were gone. My heart was much calmer and I didn't feel as if I was constantly about to go into a-fib.

I wasn't completely out of the woods yet though. Just as it can take years to develop a magnesium deficiency it can also take years to correct it. I read up about the various types of magnesium – from the virtually useless cheap magnesium oxide which is used in some supplements to more absorbable magnesium citrate and taurate. I started to use magnesium citrate and within six months my a-fib episodes had completely stopped.

Becoming complacent and thinking I was totally cured, I became lax with my magnesium. This, combined with a bad stomach bug which totally depleted my remaining minerals "rewarded" me with an 8 hour surprise a-fib attack. If ever there was proof that my a-fib was caused by mineral deficiency this was it.

I then "discovered" transdermal magnesium – a highly absorbable form of the mineral which is rubbed on the skin. I personally found this much more convenient than taking supplements by mouth, particularly as magnesium can cause loose stools and other problems when taken orally.

I take no drugs, I have had no surgery and I remain a-fib free and have for several years. I haven't seen a doctor for a-fib in 7 years now and I remain in perfect sinus rhythm.

If the doctors tell you that your a-fib occurs "for no particular reason", refuse to accept this. Turn detective, keep an a-fib diary, become familiar with the latest research and medical studies and speak to other people who have experienced a-fib. Particularly, those of us who have won our battle with it. There are a lot of us out there – and more are joining us every day.

.

---

[i] The effect of mastic gum on Helicobacter pylori: a randomized pilot study. (*Dabos KJ, Sfika E, Vlatta LJ, Giannikopoulos G.*)

[ii] (Efficacy of acupuncture in preventing atrial fibrillation recurrences after electrical cardioversion.) *Lomuscio A[1], Belletti S, Battezzati PM, Lombardi F.*

[iii] Acupuncture for paroxysmal and persistent atrial fibrillation: An effective non-pharmacological tool? *Federico Lombardi, Sebastiano Belletti, Pier Maria Battezzati, and Alberto Lomuscio*

[iv] http://www.eftuniverse.com/cardiovascular-illnesses/eft-for-atrial-fibrillation